20 DAYS TO A TRIMMER TORSO

by Cal del Pozo

Photographs by Ralph Bogertman

CORNERSTONE LIBRARY
Published by Simon & Schuster, Inc.
New York

Copyright © 1984 by Cal del Pozo
All rights reserved
including the right of reproduction
in whole or in part in any form
Published by Cornerstone Library
A Division of Simon & Schuster, Inc.
Simon & Schuster Building
1230 Avenue of the Americas
New York, New York 10020

Designed by Stanley S. Drate

CORNERSTONE LIBRARY and colophon are registered trademarks of
Simon & Schuster, Inc.
10 9 8 7 6 5 4 3 2 1
Manufactured in the United States of America
ISBN: 0-346-12588-X

700687

CAUTION:

Before starting this,
or any other exercise program,
it is advisable to check
with your physician.

FOREWORD

Have you ever wondered how dancers get to look that good? And how they stay looking that good? Well, Cal del Pozo is a dancer, and he looks that good because he, as all dancers do, spends a major portion of his life practicing one of the three imperatives of preventive medicine—exercise. The other two, in case you didn't know, are stop smoking and lose weight.

Exercise is in many ways the most difficult of the three to master for it requires you to *start* doing something rather than *stop* doing something. And Cal, in this, as in his previous books, gives you a lot to do.

None of it is magic, and not much of it is dramatically new. What is new, however, is the approach he uses: lighthearted, (occasionally lightheaded) and carefully avoiding the pompous approach of too many exercise books.

No exercise book is worth the paper it's printed on if it doesn't make the process fun—something to look forward to rather than something to dread. One of the best ways to do that is to exercise with a friend, or better yet, a spouse.

One final word of caution; if the most exercise you have gotten in the last few years is opening the refrigerator or walking to the deli for cigarettes, see your doctor before you start this or any exercise program.

So, while you are following Cal's advice and doing his exercises, stop smoking and lose weight. Your body and your doctor will thank you. Be healthy!

PAUL SCOLES, M.D.

CONTENTS

3

MORE TRIMMING TIPS

INTRODUCTION

Last fall my first book, *Bunnetics*, was released. In it I confessed to suffering from bunophobia, the fear of a drooping derriere. Since the book's release, others have tried to explore the theory behind the behind. I, though, can proudly say that thanks to your support and that of newspaper and magazine articles all across the country, not to mention radio and television programs such as "The Phil Donahue Show," I have been able to shape, trim, and lift thousands of sagging bottoms.

But, as in all true confessions, I left something out. I also suffer from torsilitis, an awful condition that can cause your torso to spread, almost overnight. Your stomach swells, your back hunches, your sides widen and slack, your shirts tear, your belts snap, and before you know it the torsilitis virus can slow down your entire body.

But no more. Through years of research and practice I have found the antidote—a series of simple home exercises coupled with some basic information about your body. Regardless of how old you are, or how sedentary you have been, or how much the effect of physical neglect or holiday eating has contributed to the environment that harbors this virus, in just TWENTY DAYS you can be rid of it forever. It's all in this book. No more tucking in when a loved one hugs you. No more bulky sweaters or black overcoats. It's your torso. You are the boss! All you need to do is spend a few minutes a day giving it some love and tender care and you will see the change. In just TWENTY DAYS, I will trim two to four inches off your waist, flatten your stomach, trim your arms, and improve your posture. You will look and feel strong, trimmed, sensuous, and healthy. Find out how simple and easy it will be. Together, we can win the fight in TWENTY DAYS.

Cal del Pozo

20 DAYS TO A TRIMMER TORSO

THE CONTENTS

In past years, good looks relied on clothes and cosmetics. Today, the trend is turning. In fact, Mother Nature is putting up a good fight and good bodies are what is knocking people off the sidewalks. No Liz Taylor eyes or Clark Gable moustaches. No Joan Crawford shoulder pads or Fred Astaire top hats. A strong body in a trimmed torso and watch out! Brooke Shields's agent might just be around the corner with contract and lagoon on hand. But Mother Nature provides only the raw materials. You and I must make the molds. So get yourself ready because we are going to chisel away. In TWENTY DAYS we have to make, bake, and polish the mold that will make your torso into a masterpiece. Impossible? Hard? No! Easy, you'll see.

BUILD A BETTER TORSO
BAKE A BETTER MOLD

You just wondered if Mother Nature gave you too much raw material. Don't let it worry you. A fabulous, trimmed, and sensuous torso can be yours in no time at all. No machines to buy or pills to take. No clubs to attend or exercise suits to wear. You want to walk around in slinky faded jeans and shrunken old sweatshirts looking great?

You can do it! Standing beside you, your Adidas-wrapped neighbor could look as fat and overdressed as a penguin in a nudist colony.

THE BLUEPRINT

20 Days to a Trimmer Torso is divided into three main sections. Part One, Mind Over Body, is a collage of resourceful information that you will find extremely beneficial to your goal. It will give you many of the answers to the common problem of a spreading torso.

Part Two contains The Centering Program. Here you will find the exercises. They are fully illustrated and their instructions are easy to follow and do. I will show you the way they should be done and tell you the way they should feel. The goals you will be striving for will be repeatedly emphasized. This section also contains the "Stretch/Strength Warm-Up" routine which you will do before each group of exercises.

Finally, in Part Three, you will find More Trimming Tips. These are a series of suggestions that you can follow throughout the day and that will speed up your progress. There you are. Three short, fun, easy-to-read-and-do sections that will pay off with looks of jealousy and admiration.

COMBINATION PACKAGE

Although such a thing as a fat skeleton does not exist, as years progress we develop different covers for our almost identical inner frames. In order for any type of exercise system to have rapid and long-lasting effect, it has to follow, as in learning to dance, a gradual pattern. This in turn has to be tailored to the individual's shape and physical capabilities.

By combining information, results achieved through gradually intensive exercise, and encouragement, I know that you will be able to trim your torso. In fact, by the time you finish this program you will not only be in better shape, you will know how to stay in shape.

BEING PUSHY

Exercising from a book can be a lonesome task. This is one of the many reasons why people buy an exercise book and just end up leafing through the pictures. Well, it's your torso that needs the work, not your fingers. But, if you are one of the millions of people who enjoy a little push, you have found the right companion. I AM PUSHY and I LOVE COMPANY. I'll be there doing the exercises right along with you. We are going to spend a few minutes a day, together, every day for twenty days. How about that for being pushy?

READY WHEN YOU ARE

I know that adding something extra to your daily schedule, even a few minutes a day, takes a little bit of preparation. You must start when you feel you are ready. But don't just say to yourself, "Perhaps today I will try some of the exercises." Believe me, you'll be wasting your time and money. Think about it. Take your time and plan when you are going to start. Then stick to it. You won't be sorry. I'll be ready whenever you are, but remember that the longer you postpone it the harder it might be. And if it must be mañana, well, I speak Spanish as well. So look down and around. In no time your present size will be waisting away. Let's get to work.

1

*MIND
OVER
BODY*

MIND OVER BODY

The torso is made up of different units. The more information your brain stores about the components of all these units, the more efficiently those units will work. This section is geared to give you such information. The few minutes it will take you to read through it will indeed help you to A TRIMMER TORSO IN TWENTY DAYS, and to KEEP IT TRIMMED.

PROMISES PROMISES!

Oh, I know you have heard similar promises. And I am sure that many of you probably have spent a great deal of time waiting for your wrinkles to disappear, your chest to change, your thighs to shrink, or your love handles to get a divorce. Promised deadlines arrived. Ankle weights rusted. Suddenly, everyone looked forward to Easter Sunday and you couldn't find a basket large enough to hide in. Well, all I can say is YOU ARE GOING TO TRIM YOUR TORSO IN TWENTY DAYS. I PROMISE!

EXERCISE

To exercise is to develop or train our muscular structure. This can be done through free hand exercise, as in this book, or through weight training. When you exercise you are basically activating the contractile mechanism of your muscles past their relaxed or resting state to various levels beyond their present working capacity. The more you exercise the higher your muscles' capacity to work.

Anaerobic and Aerobic Exercise

There is no question that the most complete way to exercise is to combine movements that build muscle strength and promote muscle tone (anaerobic exercise), such as you will find in this book, with movements that improve endurance and heart rate through cardiovascular action (aerobic), such as running, jumping rope, dancing, etc. Exercise increases the burning of energy (calories) which your body stores in the form of fat. It isn't that exercise itself burns that many calories, but what it does is to raise your metabolic rate so that your body burns more calories throughout the day. If you are in good shape, an exercise routine that combines both anaerobic and aerobic exercise three times a week can be sufficient to keep you in better health and good physical shape. But, if you are in bad shape, you would benefit much more from daily short sessions of exercise that will strengthen your muscles and prepare you to start a more intensive exercise schedule. The exercises in this book will, in addition to trimming your torso, give you more overall strength and can be used as a marvelous foundation for a more intensive program.

The exercises I have selected for you can, after completing the first two groups, be done faster and without intervals. And although doing them faster still does not place them in an aerobic category, the increased speed allows them a certain degree of aerobic phase.

Movement vs. Exercise

I am sure that you know someone who has attended exercise classes or who exercises at home. And who other than working up a sweat, developing a few aches and pains, or perhaps even losing a couple of pounds of water weight, has maintained the same unwanted shape. Usually, the reason for this is simply badly planned and thoughtless exercise. That person has been moving, not exercising.

Our muscles are as lazy as they are smart. They would rather sit home in a comfortable chair, surrounded by Godiva chocolates and Häagen-Dazs ice cream while the stereo and the television do the work.

It is up to the individual to make sure that every movement performed by his or her muscles has an increased variety of tasks. Then you'll see them get off the chair, strong, trimmed, and dying to show off. If your torso is a chair lover, get your shoes on because in TWENTY DAYS or less it is going to surprise you.

The Overload Principle

So far the only proven method to strengthen our muscles is to subject them to progressively increasing work loads within their natural range of motion. Weight lifters, for instance, might repeat the same type of exercise for a long period but will progressively increase the load of weights. Using this method and a few huffs and puffs they can go beyond the natural look and work themselves into the well-defined muscular look we see in body magazines. Dancers learn their trade and achieve technical stability through the same gradual procedure. The exercises you will be doing are devised according to the overload principle and follow the torso's natural range of motion. That is how I know you will TRIM IT IN TWENTY DAYS.

It's All in Your Head

Muscular movement is the result of a chain reaction. The message begins in your brain. At your command, it is transmitted through the nervous system to the muscles you want to move. This we all do unconsciously. Physiologists have proven that although it is not necessary to know the exact muscular function of the areas we want to move, it helps to think about the movement we are about to do before and during execution.

This is a common drawback of exercising from a book. You look at the pictures, read the instructions, and follow the directions. You are thus exercising by copy or mimic action. And although by this action you can get results, because after all you are moving your muscles, chances are they will be too long in coming to satisfy your anxiety. The reason I know you will TRIM YOUR TORSO IN TWENTY DAYS is because you are going to combine thinking with exercising. No! You are not going to levitate or think the vacuum cleaner into action. I have tried that and ended up hiring a cleaning crew to rescue me from the dust. But you are going to make your brain's little gray cells help you trim and keep you trimmed. I promise.

The Look of Love

The torso is where all the signs of age, overeating, and physical neglect are constantly exposed. We spend a great deal of time and money on our clothes, our hair, and our faces so that we can look young, appealing, and up to date. But winter doesn't last forever and with today's summer wear there is little you can hide. A TRIM TORSO is among the most sensuous parts of the anatomy and can truly change your life and appearance.

What is the point of having thinner thighs, a firm chest, or even a beautiful bottom, if halfway down your middle you are wearing a Dunkin' Donut ad? The torso is the key to the shape of other parts of the body. Put the torso in shape. Trim it. And watch how easily and beautifully everything else comes together. Your legs will look longer and your chest will be firmer. Your bottom tighter and your hips shapelier. Concentrate your efforts on your own body's natural center and see how it makes the total you the center of attraction.

TORSO, THE CENTRAL ISSUE

Just about everything has a halfway point or center. People do, too. Doctors often refer to it as the body's core but its most common name is the torso. Dancers call it the Center and to us it represents a major portion of our daily concern and training. Did you ever wonder how such skinny-looking guys could lift their ballerinas over their heads, and keep them there? A strong torso is the answer and when it comes to taking care of it, we are experts. Therefore, the name of my exercise program, which you will find in Part Two, is called The Centering Program. It is taken from the Aerobic Centering classes that I hold in New York City, which concentrates on, you guessed it, the Torso.

The exercises themselves are selected from those that have shown quick and long-lasting results with my students. Easy, fun, and great trimmers.

A Musical Instrument

The torso is a part of the trunk. It runs from the lower end of the rib cage, where the diaphragm or breathing muscle is located, to the top of the pelvic line, where it tapers in and forms that imaginary line we call the Waistline. (If yours tapers out, don't worry. It soon won't.)

Because of the torso's unique, tubelike structure it can function much like an accordion. It can contract, extend, flex, and rotate. Its numerous muscles crisscross and overlap to form the body's natural girdle. Studied and planned exercise is the only way to fully control this complicated instrument.

Age Is a Poor Excuse

I just turned forty, which is the age when the torso goes out shopping for recliners and twenty-five-inch television screens. I know I don't look my age because I work at staying young. I have people in my classes of all ages and I work them as hard as I do myself. And they don't look their age either. YOU ARE NEVER TOO OLD TO TRIM YOUR TORSO and to look and feel younger. And if you think otherwise, GIVE ME A BREAK. Let me show you how easy it is to take inches off your body and years off your present look.

The Fountain of Youth

Throughout this book I will help you to look and feel younger. Exercise is said to be the Fountain of Youth, but a Trimmer Torso is what turns the waters on. So, let's get wet.

You are not the only one. When it comes to shaping your figure, everyone has lots of doubts and questions. I have

24

chosen a few that are constantly being presented to me. Read them and I am sure you will find a lot of them in common with your own doubts.

QUESTIONS AND ANSWERS

Q *Is spot reducing really possible?*

A To reduce or shape a particular spot of the anatomy through free hand exercise is hard, or depending on the spot, often impossible. That is, unless that spot is a major unit of the body. Our body is designed to work in units, not in isolated spots.

Q *My only problem is love handles. Do I have to do all the exercises? Isn't there just one exercise for them?*

A Exclusively, one that really works? No. Love handles are the product of bad muscle tone, fat-laden muscle, and/or skin that has lost its elasticity either due to age or lack of exercise, or both. Love handles are the merging point of two muscles, the External Obliques and the Rectus Abdominis. These muscles are major units of the torso and in order to be worked the entire torso must be worked. You can twist yourself into a frenzy and all you might achieve is a sore back or a herniated disc. Fat belongs to an entire muscular unit, not just to one spot.

Q *Do I have to go on a diet while doing the exercises?*

A No. I don't believe in diets but I do believe in watching what you eat. Overweightness is not as much a problem due to what we eat as it is to how we eat. Part Three, More Trimming Tips, contains a series of suggestions that will definitely help you to curb your eating habits and reduce the amount of calories you take in throughout your twenty-day period. But, when it comes to eating, you are your best disciplinarian.

Q *Won't just doing sit-ups trim my waistline?*

A No. It might actually make it bigger. Sit-ups are by far one of the most dangerous of all the exercises that I label as hand-me-downs. The act of sitting up does not work the stomach as properly as a Torso Curl does. Which you will be doing later. In a sit-up, especially when you anchor your feet for leverage, the hip flexor muscles and the momentum created by the head and the shoulders do most of the work. Your stomach muscles are being pumped rather than strengthened. This could, as in weight lifting, contribute to making them even bigger.

Q *Will these exercises make my torso look muscular?*

A Not necessarily. Exercise converts fat-laden muscle into lean muscle, thus contributing to a trimmer look. Women, because of different chemical and hormonal compositions, can easily increase their strength fifty percent without increasing the size of the muscle. Men, in turn, can achieve muscular definition much easier once they have rid their muscle of most of its fat content. The exercises in Groups Three and Four can be used for abdominal definition.

Q *How long does each group take?*

A Between fifteen and twenty minutes for the first two days of each group. Much less as you learn the continuity.

Q The scale tells me I'm underweight but the mirror tells a different story. Why?

A Scales do lie but mirrors seldom do. Size depends on your height, frame, and amount of muscle and skin fat. Shape depends on the firmness and tone of your muscles. When you exercise you can actually put on weight and still look slimmer. Follow the mirror and forget the scale.

Q My mother and father are both gigantic. Doesn't that make my wish for a trimmer body hopeless?

A My mother can get pretty tubby too, and if I didn't combine the time spent sitting while writing with exercise, I could give Flipper a run for his money. Heredity does have a certain amount of influence but early developmental patterns such as exercise and activity do too, regardless of family size. CHANGING, especially in our adult years, the type or combination of body type we have is hard, but SHAPING IT, TRIMMING IT, and FIRMING IT is within everyone's reach. Regardless of Mom and Dad.

Q Why is it that although I jog three times a week I still have a bigger stomach than I'd like?

A Jogging is an aerobic exercise. It improves your cardio-vascular system and works your leg muscles. But, if you combine your jogging with the exercises in this book you will see an incredible change in your shape in very little time. And I mean incredible.

Q In high school I was an All-State athlete with a thirty-inch waist. Today, I still participate in sports but my waist is thirty-six and climbing. Why?

A Because the torso is a cylindrical structure by nature, it tends to constantly look for that form. When our body stops growing upward, it continues to grow outward. Most sports, including football and baseball, do not exercise the muscles of the torso to their fullest. Try swimming or handball.

Q *In my work I never stop moving and I still have a weight problem. Why?*

A Daily activity is movement which your muscles get used to and can endure with decreasing expenditure of burned energy. A few minutes a week of exercise combined with an active life and your only weight problem will be from those trying to hang on to you. But, if you exercise and eat sensibly, and still have a weight problem, you should definitely consult with your doctor.

Q *Is all this fitness craze worth it? Aren't we getting too narcissistic? What kind of example are we setting for our children? (These questions were put to me during a recent appearance on "The Phil Donahue Show.")*

A Getting in shape and staying in shape are obligations we have for the maintenance of good health. God provided us with a body as a fine instrument. Keeping it tuned is the least we can do. Good looks are just one of the benefits we derive from exercise. If we strive to stay in shape, and thus improve our looks, our children will most likely do the same. Trimming your torso is as beneficial to your health as it is to your appearance and it will just take you TWENTY DAYS TO FIND OUT.

THE MUSCLE ENGINE

Muscles, in order to be strengthened, must be made to contract (action which shortens its fibers) and to extend in alternating and continuous bursts. Contractability is one of the muscles' various characteristics, it being stronger in some than in others depending on their location and function. In the torso, muscles are able to sustain contraction for a longer period of time and are also able to support the body and protect it from shock or heavy weight—if they are in good condition.

Burning Fat

Muscles contain certain enzymes that allow them to burn calories much faster than any other tissue in the body. But fat-laden muscle cannot move with the agility of lean muscle, thus the property of these enzymes in such cases becomes inhibited. Besides, muscles that have stayed sedentary, when exercised, will rebel in the form of pain. This is the reason why more than sixty-five percent of the people who embark on exercise resolutions seldom follow them through.

My Secret

Aware of this obstacle, I have constructed my exercises to follow a gradual pattern of increasing movement. That is how I plan to get your muscle engine working without stalling. We'll start slowly but will end up full-speed ahead. TONING, FIRMING, SLIMMING, and TRIMMING IN TWENTY DAYS.

Remember that the torso is a collage of units. Thus, the trimming mechanism actually starts from deep inside. You will be trimming that torso from the first day of the exercises, but don't despair if you don't see a difference in your measurements right away. Before the first two inches can come off your waist, you have to give the muscles time to know you mean business. But by the middle of the second week you'll see what I mean. IT WILL HAPPEN. YOU WILL SEE THE DIFFERENCE. But you cannot expect to lose overnight what might have taken you a lifetime to accumulate. If you follow my instructions A TRIMMER TORSO CAN BE YOURS IN TWENTY DAYS.

The Components

These are the primary movements that form the Centering exercises. I have listed them in the order of continuity and muscle conditioning that they will maintain throughout all four groups. You will find yourself coming back to this chart quite often. It will be of invaluable help in the thought process behind the execution of the exercises.

MOVEMENTS	EXTERNAL MUSCLES	BODY AREAS
1. Torso Curls	Rectus abdominis	Upper Stomach
	Lattisimus dorsi	Middle Back
	External obliques	Center Stomach
	Sacrospinalis	Lower Back
2. Reverse Curls	Rectus abdominis	Lower Stomach
	External obliques	Sides
	Sacrospinalis	Spine
3. Opposition Curls	Rectus abdominis	Upper and Lower Stomach
	Lattisimus dorsi	Upper Back and Sides
	External obliques	Middle Back, Lower Sides
	Sacrospinalis	Spine
	Serratus anterior	Upper Sides
4. Side Bends	Lattisimus dorsi	Sides
	External obliques	Sides
	Serratus anterior	Sides
	Trapezius	Sides, Upper and Middle Back
5. Back Bends	All muscles	

More Benefits from a Trimmer Torso

In Terms of Health:
1. Better respiration, circulation, and digestion.
2. More vitality, ability to relax and to cope with daily stress and muscular tightness.
3. More flexibility and protection from injury to the neck, back, vital organs, and lower back pain.
4. Increased stamina and better sexual performance.
5. Women who have good abdominal muscle tone are known to have easier childbirths and faster recovery rates.

In Terms of Appearance:
1. You will look younger, more rested, confident, and radiant.
2. Better posture.
3. Better muscle tone, balance, and coordination.

In Terms of Money Savings:
1. No tailoring bills.
2. A wider selection of ready-made clothes to buy.
3. Fewer visits to the doctor.

2

THE CENTERING PROGRAM

2

THE
GATHERING
PROGRAM

THE CENTERING PROGRAM

Now that you know as much (perhaps even more) about the torso and its structure as Michelangelo, let's do what the master was never able to accomplish. Trim Torsos in Twenty Days. And even though his beautiful, sculptured torsos have been and will continue to be in good shape for a long time, I can guarantee that you will have more fun with yours.

DANCE ANYONE?

Dancers refer to the torso as the Center. For us the Center greatly determines the success of our performances. It is the area where during movement all the balancing and coordinating forces of the body meet. But you don't have to join the Robert Joffrey Ballet or dance with Juliet Prowse in order to shape up. This book is all you will need to see those belt notches disappear right into your Swan Lake dreams. Whether you want to lift your spouse in an overhead split or have that Loni Anderson waist, all you need is to spend a few minutes a day with me for TWENTY DAYS.

TWENTY DAYS—TRIM AWAY AND DANCE AWAY!

The exercises you are about to do have been selected from my Aerobic Centering exercise classes in New York

City. The exercises are divided into four groups and follow a set pattern.

TAKING INCHES OFF

Each group is spread over a five-day period and works as the toning, conditioning, and trimming basis for the group that follows it. Simply, slowly grinding two to four inches away and effortlessly developing a trimmer torso.

The first group, the Basic Group, is designed to get you started. It is simple and easy and it will put you on the road to STRENGTHEN and TONE the torso area. The second group, the Intermediate Exercises, starts the FIRMING process. The third group, the Advanced Exercises, continues this process and starts to show the TRIMMING effects. And finally, the fourth group, which I call the Final Combination, ROUNDS OUT and SOLIDIFIES your goal and becomes your tailor-made exercise routine for the maintenance of your beautifully trimmed torso.

THE NATURAL WAY

When we get out of shape we do so slowly. To get in shape, and stay in shape, we must follow the same natural course. Thus, all five exercises follow a set pattern of gradual strengthening and muscular conditioning through natural body actions. They consist of flexion, extension, and rotation. These are also natural functions of the torso.

In addition, the exercises are planned according to the requirements for the development of muscle strength and tone, and the elimination of muscular fat. These are isometric and isotonic contraction. Furthermore, most of the movements use the force of gravity as resistance much in the same manner exercise machines work (isokinetic).

THE FIXED POINT

In all the exercises the movements must be thought of as starting from the center of the stomach or FIXED POINT. Think of this point as an imaginary band that circles the torso and starts and ends on your belly button. You must always CONCENTRATE ON THIS POINT BEFORE AND DURING the exercises. Doing this will add rhythm, control, and improve the alignment of your movements. These three factors are the key to successful and productive exercising.

HOW TO FOLLOW YOUR PROGRESS

Each group contains five exercises. Each exercise is illustrated according to starting or Preparation position and execution or Action. Under each exercise there is a Progression Chart (PC). Each day is noted by the letter D, and followed by a number, which tracks your progression. (Example: Day One = D1, Day Four = D4.)

The Progression Chart will also tell you the number of times an exercise should be done on that day. [Example: Day One (D1) Four Times (4×), Day Three (D3) Six Times (6×)]. There is a place indicated by parentheses [()], where you can check (/) as you finish the repetitions suggested for that day. This is how it will look:

PC:D1–2× (   ), D2–4× (   ), D3–6× (   ), D4–8× (   ), D5–10× (   )

Remember: "DAYS LOST = INCHES NOT LOST"

FOR FASTER RESULTS WITH LESS EFFORT

1. Check a calendar. Select a twenty-day period free of long interruptions such as holidays, birthday parties, long weekend vacations. Avoid obstacles. You'll have plenty of time to show off your new slinky look. What could be more fun?

2. It is always better to exercise on a rug or thinly padded mat.

3. Wear loose-fitting or exercise attire.

4. Keep handy a small hand towel that you can place under the end of your spine when doing curling moves. It will act as a small cushion and will protect you from skin irritation in this area.

5. Get a tape measure and write down your torso's measurements at the beginning of each exercise group. Measure: Chest (under breast line); Torso (under rib cage line); Waist (slightly above the belly button); and Lower Abdomen (slightly above hip bone line). You'll find a place to do this before each group.

6. Follow the Progression Chart. All the exercises are constructed with a purpose, a trimmer torso in twenty days, gradually, safely, and efficiently.

READY? PLAN YOUR SCHEDULE NOW AND IN TWENTY DAYS, WOW!

THE ARTISTS AND THE MECHANICS

When it comes to exercise I divide people into two groups: the artists and the mechanics. The first group allows time to be in the correct position, thinks of what they are doing, and tries to keep form, rhythm, and continuity. They are artistic and their efforts pay off over a long period but continuous time.

The second group, the mechanics, just goes full force right from the start. They go through the motions and want to get the work over quickly. They don't take time to think. They just do it and want to get results fast. They also lose interest, fast. Both groups will see results in twenty days but only one group will keep them. Easy comes, easy goes. Which group would you rather belong to? Remember that the key to productive exercise is in how you are exercising.

OVERWEIGHT

No one knows better than yourself if you are overweight. Statistics show that over fifty-five percent of Americans are, so you are not alone. But if at the present time you find you are more than fifteen pounds overweight, I would recommend you start by just doing the exercises in the first two groups, the Basic and the Intermediate, until you lose some of that weight. In Part Three, you'll find additional trimming tips that will help you to shed some pounds. Remember that exercise alone is not the answer. But you know that, don't you?

DOCTOR'S ADVICE

If you have not exercised in a long time you should always consult with your physician before you do. Take this book to him and show him what it is you will be doing. I have several doctors in my exercise classes and they know how your present physical state can respond to excessive movement. Especially if you suffer from back pain or high blood pressure. Always play it safe.

BREATHING

Proper breathing is the most important factor in correct exercise. When you breathe properly you are sending oxygenated blood to the areas you are working on. You'll be able to work longer and with less chance of fatigue or muscle cramps. Proper breathing is emphasized in all the exercises and should follow the following rules:

1. Inhale through the nose and exhale through the mouth.

2. Inhale while you are thinking of the movement you are about to do. Blood will flow to that area faster.

3. Exhale as you are executing the most difficult part of the movement.

4. Proper inhalation is felt when you feel the air reach down into your stomach and fill the abdominal cavity.

5. Proper exhalation is felt as the lower stomach and abdominal cavity caves in. In both, exhalation and inhalation, the chest should be free of tension.

6. Take at least twice as long to exhale as you did to inhale.

THE STRETCH/STRENGTH WARM-UP

The following movements should be done every day before starting your five-day group. They will get your muscles and your thinking processes ready. You will also find them beneficial to releasing muscle tightness after sleeping, and stress accumulated from a day's routine.

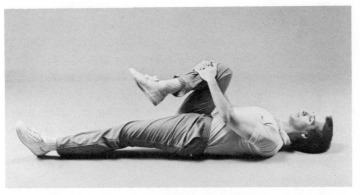

PICTURE A

PICTURE A. **Step One:** Lie back as I am doing. Body should be fully extended in a straight line and relaxed. Take a deep breath and bring one knee to your chest. Exhale slowly as you bring the knee closer to the chest. **Step Two:** Repeat with other knee.

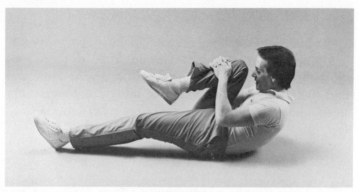

PICTURE B

PICTURE B. **Step One:** Hold starting knee again. Inhale deeply. Concentrate on your center (FIXED POINT). As you exhale curl the torso upward, bringing your forehead as close to the knee as possible. Remember that the curling action starts from the FIXED POINT. Once there, release the knee and slowly return to starting position. Lower back first, then middle, upper, and head is last. **Step Two:** Do the same for the other side.

PICTURE C. **Step One:** Inhale. Without holding onto the knee bring both forehead and knee as close as possible. Once there, HOLD THE POSITION AS YOU EXHALE SLOWLY. Notice that the arms are kept extended forward and slightly off the floor. Now return to starting position as you inhale. **Step Two:** Repeat with the other side.

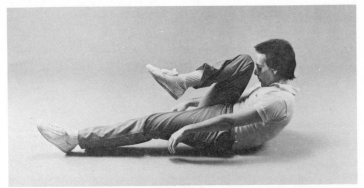

PICTURE C

PICTURE D. **One Step Only:** Inhale, then as you exhale bring both knees and forehead together. Hold the position with your arms and try to stay in that position for a few seconds. Breathe evenly. Now you are ready for your daily group.

Note: If you have tight back muscles, do the above warm-up a few times during the day to release that tension.

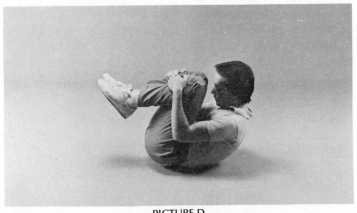

PICTURE D

GROUP ONE—BASIC EXERCISES

Measure:
Chest_____
Torso_____
Waist_____
Lower Abdomen_____

Exercise #1

Basic Two-Way Curl (Pictures 1 and 2)

Preparation: Lie back with hands clasped under your head. Knees bent and no farther apart than width of hip bone. Feet as close to the pelvis as possible. Keep knees bent at a 90° angle.

Action One (Picture 1): Inhale. Exhale as you tuck your stomach in. The point at which you see my hand is the FIXED POINT. Feel the lower back get closer to the floor. Now raise the buttocks off the floor as if you are trying to fold your pelvis over my hand. Then inhale as you place the buttocks down. Follow immediately with Action Two.

Action Two (Picture 2): Exhale as you bring chin to chest and continue to curl upward until your shoulder blades are off the floor. Don't use your elbows for momentum. Inhale as you roll back down. Both actions count as one time (1x).

PC: D1–2x(*), D2—4x ( ), D3–6x ( ), D4–8x ( ), D5–10x ( ).

*See p. 37 for explanation of Progression Chart.

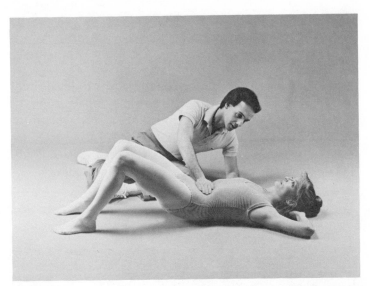

PICTURE 1

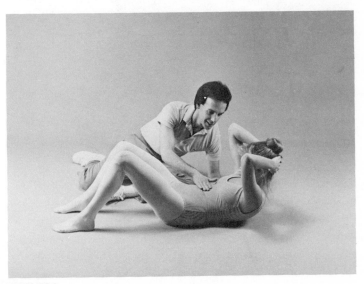

PICTURE 2

45

Exercise #2

Basic Knee Raise (Picture 3)

Preparation: Place arms alongside of body with knees bent and feet as close to the pelvis as possible. Inhale.

Action: Exhale as you bring your knees over your torso UNTIL YOU FEEL YOUR BUTTOCKS HAVE CLEARED THE FLOOR. Remember this action starts from the Fixed Point. Inhale as you place the feet back on the floor. Slowly.

PC: D1–2x ( ), D2–4x ( ), D3–6x ( ), D4–8x ( ), D5–10x ( ).

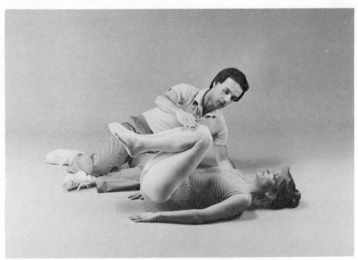

PICTURE 3

Exercise #3

Basic Opposition Twist (Picture 4)

Preparation: Lie back with body fully extended and arms to the side. Inhale.

Action One: Exhale. Lift leg and opposite arm. Reach over to the leg. Notice how the head maintains the tucked chin in position. Inhale as you return to starting position.

Action Two: Repeat same with the other arm and leg. Both actions constitute 1x.

PC: D1–2x ( ), D2–4x ( ), D3–6x ( ), D4–8x ( ), D5–10x ( ).

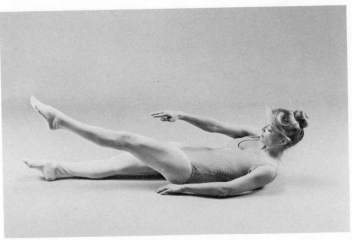

PICTURE 4

Exercise #4

Basic Side Bend (Pictures 5 and 6)

Preparation: As in Picture 5, make sure that the extended leg forms a straight line with the torso and the arm that is placed under the head. Inhale.

Action (Picture 6): Lift the side of the body off the floor as you exhale. Feel the upper hand reach down the upper thigh. Inhale on the way down. Roll over and do the other side. Look at the PC before starting. Remember it is for both sides.

PC: D1–1x ( ), D2–2x ( ), D3–3x ( ), D4–4x ( ), D5–5x ( ).

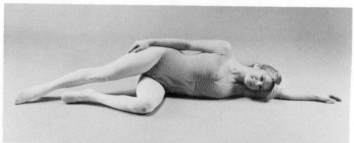

PICTURE 5

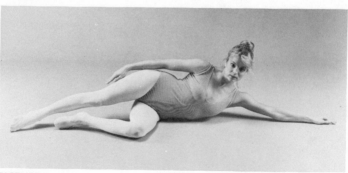

PICTURE 6

Exercise #5

Basic Back Bend (Pictures 7 and 8)

Preparation: As in Picture 7, lie face down and open arms in a wide V. Inhale.

Action (Picture 8): As you exhale, lift the torso off the floor as far down as the lower rib cage. Inhale on the way down and start again. Follow the PC.

PC: D1–2x ( ), D2–2x ( ), D3–3x ( ), D4–4x ( ), D5–5x ( ).

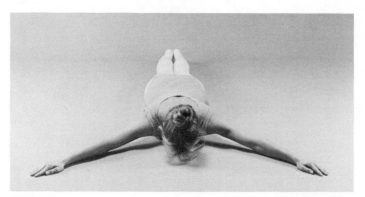

PICTURE 7

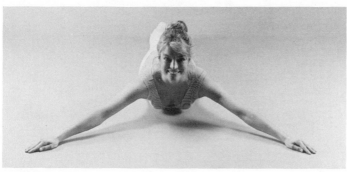

PICTURE 8

Note: With the completion of this five-day group you have started the strengthening and toning of your torso. As you see, it was easy. The next two groups are simple variations of the first group. You will find that as you progress you will develop better timing and both your execution and breathing rhythm will become second nature.

GROUP TWO—INTERMEDIATE EXERCISES

Measure:
Chest_____
Torso_____
Waist_____
Lower Abdomen_____

Exercise #1

Intermediate Two-Way Curl (Pictures 9 and 10)

Preparation: Back lying position with arms alongside the body. Knees bent and feet as close to the pelvis as possible.
Action One (Picture 9): Inhale. Exhale and lift the pelvis up until you form a straight line from your knees down to the beginning of the shoulder blades. DO NOT USE PRESSURE AGAINST THE FLOOR WITH THE FEET TO LIFT UP. Inhale on the way down. Follow immediately with Action Two.

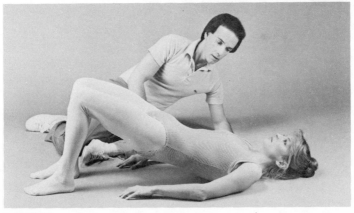

PICTURE 9

Action Two (Picture 10): Exhale as you curl the torso. Arms off the floor and reaching down toward the feet. Both actions constitute 1x.

PC: D1–3x ( ), D2–6x ( ), D3–9x ( ), D4–12x ( ), D5–15x ( ).

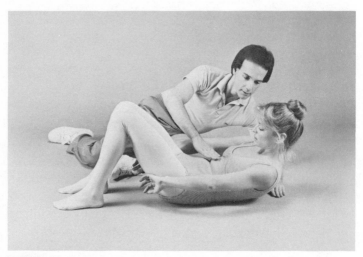

PICTURE 10

Exercise #2

Intermediate Knee Raise (Picture 11)

Preparation: Back lying position with knees bent and arms resting alongside of body. Inhale.

Action: Exhale as you curl the upper torso and the knees toward each other. Arms come off the floor and reach straight ahead. Inhale as you roll down.

PC: D1–3x ( ), D2–6x ( ), D3–9x ( ), D4–12x ( ), D5–15x ( ).

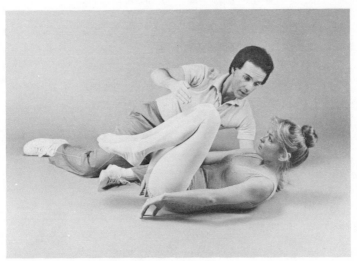

PICTURE 11

Exercise #3

Intermediate Twist (Pictures 12–14)

Preparation (Picture 12): Back lying position with hands clasped behind the head. Inhale.

Action One (Picture 13): Exhale quickly as you bring opposite elbow and knee together. Inhale as you lower the knee and roll down to preparation position.

Action Two (Picture 14): Now do the same with the other knee and elbow. Each action counts as 1x.

PC: D1–6x ( ), D2–10x ( ), D3–14x ( ), D4–20x ( ), D5–26x ( ).

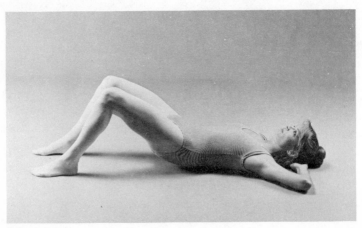

PICTURE 12

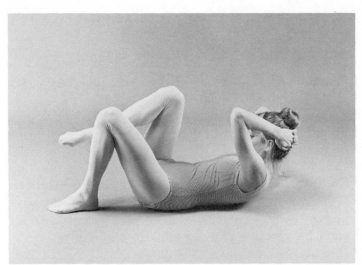

PICTURE 13

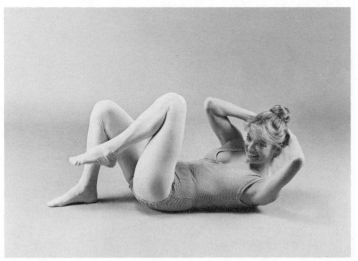

PICTURE 14

Exercise #4

Intermediate Side Bend (Picture 15)

Preparation: This time lie on one side BUT WITH LEGS FULLY EXTENDED. Inhale.

Action (Picture 15): Exhale as you raise upper body off the floor. Inhale on the way down. Roll over and do the same on the other side.

Note: Keeping the legs extended makes it a little harder to keep from rolling the body forward or backward. That is just the point. Concentrate on keeping your balance and you'll be trimming a lot more than just the side muscles.

PC: D1–4x ( ), D2–6x ( ), D3–8x ( ), D4–10x ( ), D5–12x ( ).

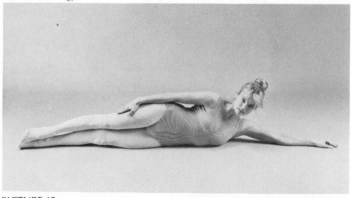

PICTURE 15

Exercise #5

Intermediate Back Bend (Picture 16)

Preparation: Lie face down and clasp hands behind the head. Inhale.

Action (Picture 16): Exhale as you lift torso off the floor. Keep feet down. Inhale on way down. Remember to do it slowly.

PC: D1–4x ( ), D2–6x ( ), D3–8x ( ), D4–10x ( ), D5–12x ( ).

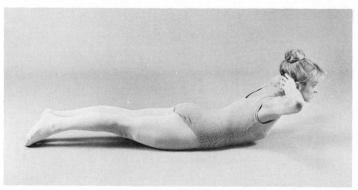

PICTURE 16

Note: Upon completion of your five-day Intermediate Group you should already feel and see a difference in your torso. This is really the no-turn-back point. You have come halfway and it is from here that you will see an upward trend in your trimming process. Your friends will see it too. Ten more days and you can send your picture to the "Dynasty" series casting office. Remember me if they call you back.

GROUP THREE—ADVANCED EXERCISES

A Warning About Skipping

As simple as the following exercises look, doing them without having executed the two previous groups could bring unwanted muscle cramps and pains UNLESS YOU ARE A PERSON WHO ALREADY ENGAGES IN A WEEKLY EXERCISE ROUTINE.

MEN looking for abdominal muscle definition, trimmer love handles, and a smaller waistline and WHO HAVE EXERCISED REGULARLY will find the next two groups perfect for achieving those goals. Doubling the doses suggested in the PC, with small periods of rest in between, will further those goals even more.

Measure:
Chest_____
Torso_____
Waist_____
Lower Abdomen_____

Exercise #1

Advanced Full Curl (Pictures 17 and 18)

Preparation (Picture 17): Lie back and wrap arms over torso. Men wrap over chest. Women wrap under breast line. Inhale.

Action (Picture 18): Exhale as you feel the curling motion start from the FIXED POINT. Stop as you feel the last lumbar vertebrae leave the floor (approximately 45° off the floor). This is the point where the force of gravity and the muscle's contracting fibers cooperate for maximum result. Inhale and roll down.

PC: D1–10x ( ), D2–15x ( ), D3–20x ( ), D4–25x ( ), D5–30x ( ).

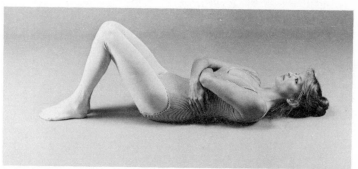

PICTURE 17

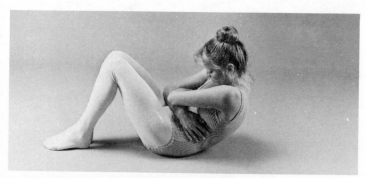

PICTURE 18

Exercise #2

Advanced Knee Raise (Pictures 19–22)

Preparation (Picture 19): Lie back with knees bent and together. Feet as close to pelvis as possible and arms alongside the body. Inhale.

Action One (Picture 20): Exhale as you curl lower abdomen up and bring knees over to your right side. COUNT ONE. Keep shoulder blades on the floor.

Action Two (Picture 21): Inhale as you extend legs straight ahead off the floor about 40°. Keep arms and lower back firmly against the floor. COUNT TWO.

Action Three (Picture 22): Exhale as you bring knees over to the other side. COUNT THREE. Inhale as you extend the legs off the floor again. COUNT FOUR. All four counts constitute one set (1s).

PC: D1–5s ( ), D2–5s ( ), D3–10s ( ), D4–10s ( ), D5–10s ( ).

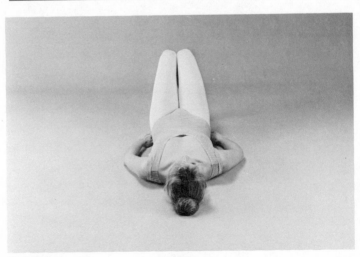

PICTURE 19

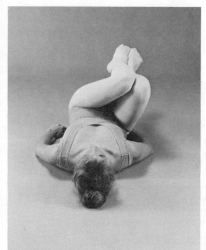

PICTURE 20

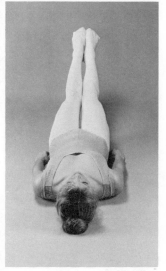

PICTURE 21

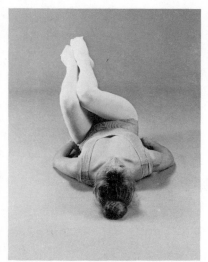

PICTURE 22

Exercise #3

Advanced Continuous Twist (Pictures 23 and 24)

This is a fast-paced endurance exercise that requires you to inhale and exhale through the mouth with rapid action.

Preparation: Bring both feet off the floor, knees bent and parallel, and keep hands clasped behind the head. Lift torso to half-curl position.

Action (Picture 23): Exhale and bring right elbow and left knee toward each other. (Picture 24) Inhale quickly and repeat action with opposites as you exhale. Keep the actions quick and rhythmical. Each twist counts as 1x.

PC: D1–20x ( ), D2–20x ( ), D3–20x ( ), D4–30x ( ), D5–30x ( ).

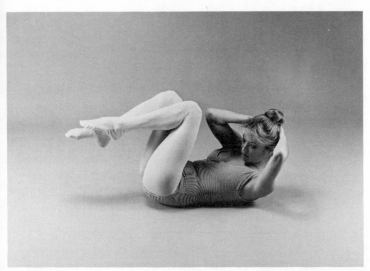

PICTURE 23

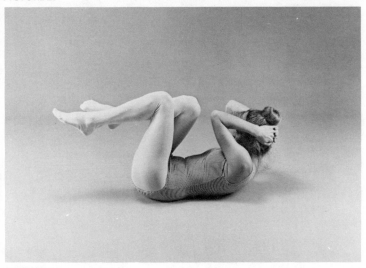

PICTURE 24

Exercise #4

Advanced Side Bend (Pictures 25 and 26)

Preparation: As in Picture 25, lie on one side. Bring knees toward chest. Place one hand on the floor, and in front of waistline, with fingers pointing toward your head. The other arm is extended under the head. Inhale.

Action (Picture 26): Exhale as you push with your hand against the floor and at the same time try to move lower shoulder and upper knee to meet. Return to preparation position as you exhale. Repeat with the other side.

PC: D1–5x ( ), D2–8x ( ), D3–10x ( ), D4–12x ( ), D5–15x ( ).

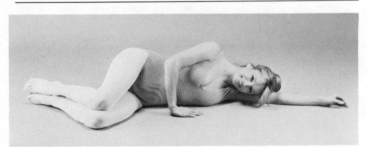

PICTURE 25

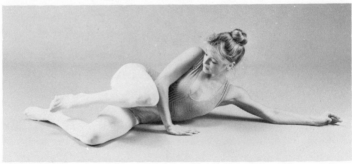

PICTURE 26

Exercise #5

Advanced Back Bend (Picture 27)

Preparation: Lie face down with hands clasped behind the head. Inhale.

Action (Picture 27): Exhale as you lift torso up and extend arms to the side and outward forming a V. Lie down again as you inhale.

PC: D1–6x ( ), D2–6x ( ), D3–8x ( ), D4–10x ( ), D5–10x ( ).

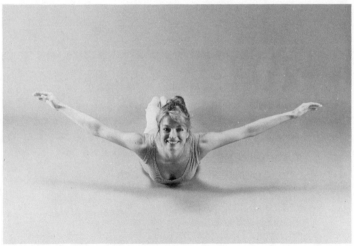

PICTURE 27

GROUP FOUR—FINAL COMBINATION

This is the level you have so diligently worked for. I know that if you have followed the progression of your groups you must be very excited by your measurements. This group will carry you even further along. I call it the Final Combination because it brings together the best, safest, and most proven movements to round out your exercise program and to help you keep a TRIMMER TORSO BEYOND YOUR TWENTY-DAY GOAL.

Measure:
Chest_____
Torso_____
Waist_____
Lower Abdomen_____

Exercise #1

Sit-Up Combination (Pictures 28–31)

Preparation: As in Picture 28, lie on the floor with legs together and arms to the side and outward.

Action One (Picture 29): Exhale. As you do a Full Curl, wrap both arms around your upper chest. COUNT ONE.

Action Two (Picture 30): Inhale as you roll down to Half Curl position. Arms will move down to lower torso. Keep arms in wrapped position. COUNT TWO.

Action Three (Picture 31): Exhale as you sit up and extend legs forward, and arms straight up. Keep back and neck in a straight line. COUNT THREE. Inhale as you roll back down to preparation position. COUNT FOUR. All four counts constitute one set (1s).

PC· Ten full sets every time.

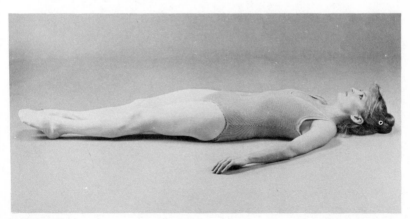

PICTURE 28 ⟶

67

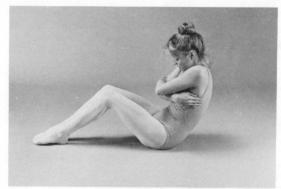

PICTURE 29

PICTURE 30

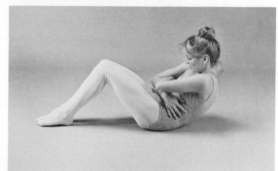

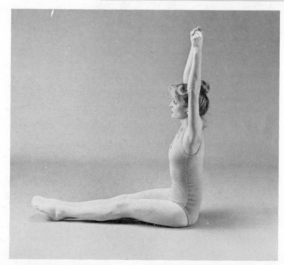

PICTURE 31

Exercise #2

Knee Raise Combination (Pictures 32 and 33)

Preparation: As in Picture 32, start with legs straight, toes pointed and about one foot off the floor. As you lift the legs straight, concentrate on keeping the FIXED POINT close to the floor. Inhale.

Action (Picture 33): Exhale as you bring both the knees and the elbows together. Keep chin tucked in. Notice that lower and middle back remain on the floor. COUNT ONE. Inhale as you go back to starting position. COUNT TWO. Both counts constitute one set (1s).

PC: D1–4s ( ), D2–8s ( ), D3–12s ( ), D4–16s ( ), D5–20s ( ).

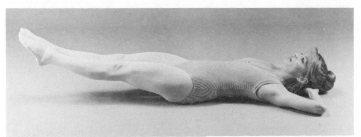

PICTURE 32

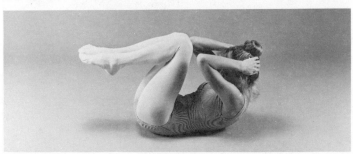

PICTURE 33

Exercise #3

Combination Twist (Pictures 34 and 35)

Preparation (Picture 34): Lie back with hands on your stomach. Keep knees bent, feet turned out and opened in a V. Inhale.

Action (Picture 35): Exhale. Sit up and twist body in one direction. Thrust arms in direction of twist. Inhale as you roll down and bring hands back to waist. Each twist counts as 1x.

PC: D1–20x ( ), D2–20x ( ), D3–30x ( ), D4–40x ( ), D5–50x ( ).

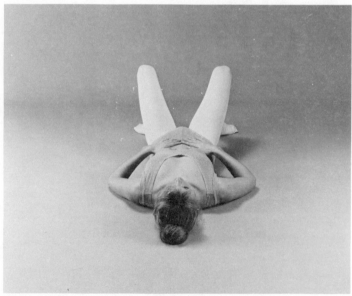

PICTURE 34

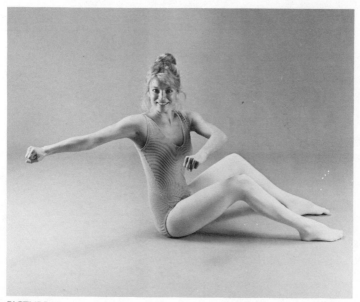

PICTURE 35

Exercise #4

Lateral Push-Up (Pictures 36 and 37)

Preparation: As in Picture 36, lie on one side and bring both thighs to a 90° angle with torso. Lower arm is folded in front of the body and upper arm is pressing against the floor. Keep the fingers pointing toward your head. Inhale.

Action (Picture 37): Exhale. Push upper body away from the floor and at the same time extend upper leg down and out. Folded arm also extends out to form a straight line with torso and extended leg. This is an extremely complete exercise and one that needs a little practice. Repeat on other side.

PC: D1–5x ( ), D2–10x ( ), D3–10x ( ), D4–10x ( ), D5–10x ( ).

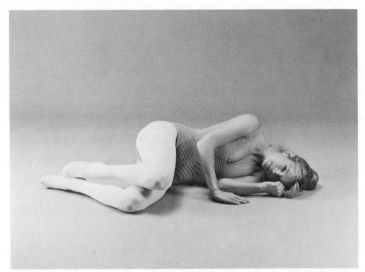

PICTURE 36

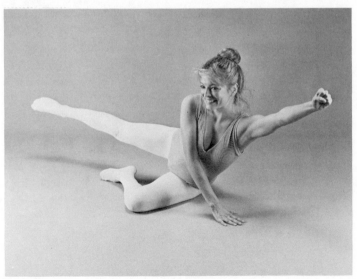

PICTURE 37

73

Exercise #5

Back Bend Combination (Pictures 38 and 39)

Preparation: As in Picture 38, lie face down with hands behind neck. Inhale.

Action (Picture 39): Exhale as you lift torso up and then twist. At the same time extend one arm back and the other forward as in a swimming position. Inhale and return to starting position. Then do the same on the other side. Each twist motion counts as 1x.

PC: Ten times every day.

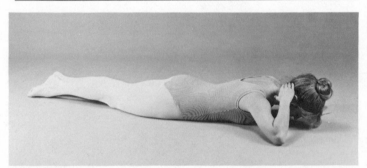

PICTURE 38

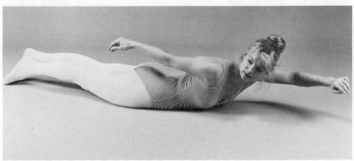

PICTURE 39

3

MORE TRIMMING TIPS

MORE TRIMMING TIPS

As much as they hate to admit it, muscles know that exercise is the only way for them to be lean, strong, and healthy. They also know that much of their beauty is always hidden by too much fat, skin, and clothing. So, let's be frank. Can you blame them if they don't particularly care for exercise? What is the point of all the work if we continue to cover them up? Mind you, I am not advocating total nudity, but is giving them a new wardrobe that difficult or expensive? Of course not!

This section will help you to do just that. More Trimming Tips will provide you with various suggestions on how to bring those muscles from the depths of the body's stockroom to the front window. It is just a matter of using a little discipline with our daily eating and physical habits. Use these tips throughout your twenty-day molding and baking spree. Turn that bisque look into a radiant and glowing piece of ceramic.

You will see how easy it is to reduce your caloric intake, the only way to reduce the fire and still come out with a perfect mold. And without having to go on starvation diets. You will also learn a few exercises that you can do while sitting at the office or standing by your desk as well as some tips on developing good posture and walking habits. Try them; they are simple.

DIETS ARE A BORE

Unless you are on a medically supervised plan because of weight problems caused by other than just too much eating, being on a diet is a boring waste of time. The amount of time spent in frustration over what you are told you can't eat, I feel, can be better spent in learning simple tips about balancing what you do eat.

When you either have too much weight or are putting on weight too rapidly there are certain things that you definitely should not do. But these are few. And seldom do any of them call for total deprivation of what makes you or your taste buds happy. Besides, thinking about going on a diet is like thinking about quitting smoking. The more you think the more you smoke.

We all know that in order to live we need to eat and that the energy food provides us with is measured in calories. The amount of exercise you do determines how much of that energy you burn and how much of it stays in the form of fat in your body. And as I said earlier, fat is found everywhere in our body. We need it. What we don't need is an overabundance of it. Balancing your caloric consumption through proper nutrition and eating habits, with your daily caloric expenditure through exercise, remains to date the only solution to a healthier and better functioning you.

But, during our twenty-day program I don't want you to be on a diet. In fact, I want you to eat. I'd much rather see you exercise than starve because I know from my own experience, and that of many of my students, that doing both at once seldom works. I have no way of knowing if you are overweight or not, but I do know that you are human. And when it comes to exercising and dieting, one of the two is going to suffer. And it usually is exercise.

So eat! You have made a smart move by starting an exercise routine that will not only trim your torso but will give you many other benefits, as well. Continue to be smart. Eat, just watch what you eat. The following tips should help you to reduce and to balance your caloric intake by developing a more discriminating eye.

SMART EATING

1. Eat whenever you FEEL hungry. Not when you THINK you are hungry. If you are nervous, open up a window and let out a scream. If you have nothing to do, take a walk. But these are THINKING-EATING REASONS not FEELING-EATING REASONS.

2. Force yourself to have breakfast. Even coffee and toast is better than nothing at all.

3. If you are a habitual snacker, great! Your metabolism is working for you all day. Just don't work it with sweets such as pastries, candies, ice creams, etc. Snack on fruits and vegetables. Look at a piece of cantaloupe and tell yourself it is a banana split. It might even taste like one.

4. Get yourself a pocket calorie book and find out how many fruits and vegetables you can snack on all day. The assortment is tremendous.

5. If you must have a dessert, have it. But then just have the dessert and not a meal with your dessert.

6. Try having JUST ONE FULL, well-balanced MEAL A DAY.

7. In full meals avoid any kind of doubling.
For instance:
If you have a potato, make it your only starch.

If you like lots of dressing in your salad, don't put any
butter or sauce on your potato.

If you are having meat for a main course, don't have any
kind of meat for an appetizer. Same for fish or fowl.

If you are having an alcoholic drink before a full meal,
have water—not wine—with your meal.

If you are having a dessert rich in sugar (few aren't),
enjoy it first, then hate yourself afterward. But at least
skip the sugar in the coffee and the after-dinner li-
queur.

8. Don't mix dairy products in any one meal or snack. Ice
cream is the best example. The fact that most brands are
made with cream *and* eggs is bad enough. Don't make it
worse by adding whipped cream.

9. When possible, broil or bake meats. But don't mix. If
you have BROILED fish don't add FRIED potatoes.

10. MOST IMPORTANT. If you must have ONE FULL
MEAL less than two hours before going to sleep, or after
ten in the evening, convince yourself either to SKIP THE
FOLLOWING DAY'S FULL MEAL (but, remember to eat
breakfast), or DO NOT EAT ANOTHER FULL MEAL FOR
TWENTY-FOUR HOURS. Snack. Skipping a meal won't kill
you.

A Step Further

If you are among the very few who make resolutions and
can stick to them, the following steps will help you even
further. As for myself, I stay with the not so strong majority.

1. Stay away from too much lamb, bacon, ham, or
sausage, as well as from luncheon processed meat. The
leaner the meat the trimmer the torso.

2. Keep to a minimum of vegetables with a high-carbo-hydrate content such as sweet potatoes and yams; beans such as kidney, lima, dried, black or red; corn; and artichokes.

3. Avoid an excess of bananas, figs, prunes, mangoes, apples, pears, pineapples, grapes, and blueberries.

4. Avoid an excess of bread (the worst—any kind), cookies (second worst), and cakes (third and most irresistible worst).

5. If you can help it, avoid beer, wine, and mixed drinks. If you are going to drink, drink straight or on the rocks. BUT NOT BEFORE MY EXERCISES, PLEASE.

THE SITTING TRIMMERS

If you spend a great deal of your time sitting, here are a few exercises that will help trim your torso while sitting.

The Basic Tuck

If you are sitting on a chair, let your head and shoulders slump forward. Keep your arms hanging loosely from the shoulders and to the sides of the chair. Think of your belly button and pull it in. Tighten it as hard as you can and count slowly up to twenty. Relax the contraction and do it again. The tighter the better. Try doing it a couple of times an hour.

The Advanced Tuck

Here's a variation of the Basic Tuck. Do one Basic Tuck and relax. Now take a real deep breath and start by tightening the stomach one more time, but this time continue the tightening contraction up the front of your body as you exhale until you are sitting straight up and you feel your back totally straight and flat. Take a deep breath while you keep this erect position and once again tighten your stomach and exhale. Keep tightening for twenty counts (approximately twenty seconds). Relax, slump forward, and repeat.

Here's Another

(Picture 40) Sit on a chair and place your hands on its seat. Keep your arms and back straight but let your head slump down. Inhale, and slowly as you exhale, pull the stomach in and bring your knees as close to the chest as possible. Inhale and place the feet on the floor again. Repeat at least fifteen times every couple of hours.

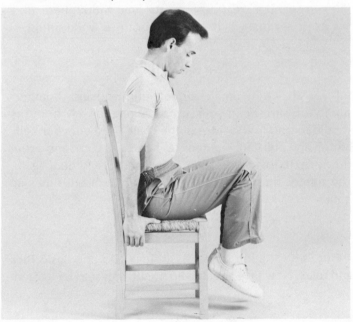

PICTURE 40

This One Is a Winner

(Picture 41) Inhale. As you exhale cross one thigh over the other and twist the opposite shoulder over to the thigh. With your hand try to reach the spot where your thigh was before you crossed it. Keep the stomach tight but the arm relaxed and hold this position for just a few seconds. Inhale and do the same with the other side. Repeat ten times whenever no one is watching.

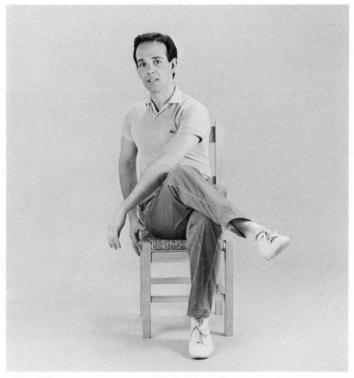

PICTURE 41

But This One Finishes the Job

(Picture 42) Sit up straight and let the arms hang to the sides. Inhale. Exhale as you reach down to the floor. (As you feel your torso bend sideways keep trying to sit tall. Don't let the sides of the body collapse as you reach.) Inhale as you straighten and repeat on the other side. Try to do at least twenty on each side a few times throughout the day.

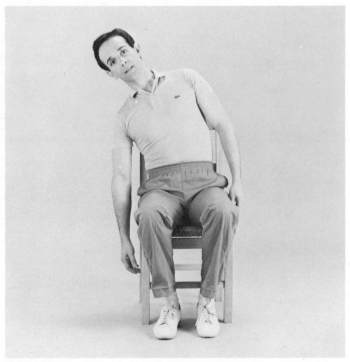

PICTURE 42

THE STANDING TRIMMERS

The Metronome

(Picture 43A) Stand straight with feet slightly apart and hands on your waist. Now bend repeatedly to both sides. (Picture 43B) What makes this common exercise really effective is not to think of bending at the waist but of concentrating on elongating one side over the other while keeping a feeling of tallness through the spine as it flexes sideways (sort of an inverted pendulum).

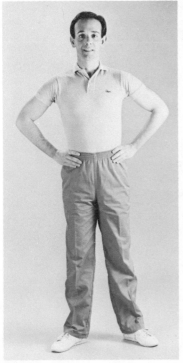

PICTURE 43A

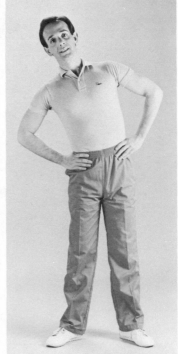

PICTURE 43B

The Low Punch

(Picture 44) Extend one arm across the body in the direction of your side bend. Feel that the arm's power of extension starts from the shoulder blades. Punch away from side to side at least twenty times.

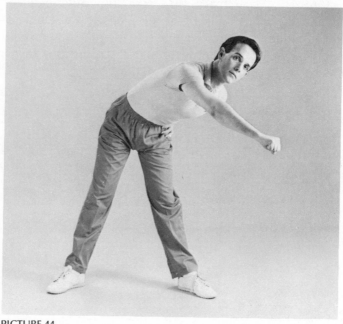

PICTURE 44

Cross Points

(Picture 45) This one will round up the major muscle groups into one final tightening action and will give your cardiovascular system a nice boost. Place your hands behind the neck. Keep elbows in line with the shoulders and bend the torso forward. Now, simultaneously, bring one elbow down to meet the knee from the opposite side. Then straighten up. Shift weight and do the same with the other knee and elbow. Try twenty counts (two on each side) to start with and each week add another ten for a grand total of fifty in your final week.

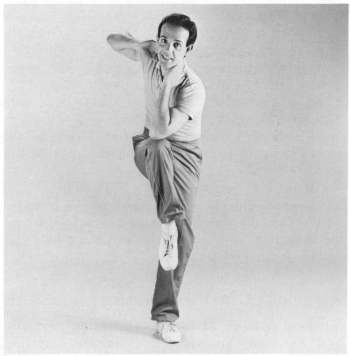

PICTURE 45

BETTER POSTURE

Give me a trimmed torso that is held tall and proud during a graceful and natural walk and I'll bet you the bearer of it has an address book the size of the New York telephone directory. Unfortunately, you don't see too many people with such torsos and good posture, which is even more fortunate for those who have it. Well, pardon me for being conceited, but I have it. And so can you.

Poor posture is the result of a combination of many elements. But contrary to popular opinion, lack of muscle tone and muscular strength are not the primary causes. Here are some of the main reasons: poor knowledge of body mechanics, an individual's profession, sleeping habits, incorrect skeletal alignment, muscle tightness due to excess stress, and the inability to relax. (All of these elements and how to improve them are covered in detail in another one of my books, *The Back Book*).

As the exercises in this book will contribute to better abdominal strength and support of the center of the body, better postural alignment will be easier to obtain. But only through simple practice and conscious thought will better posture become a daily habit.

As a matter of fact, strengthening and toning the torso's units without thought to correct posture can make bad posture more prominent. As the muscles become stronger they are able to work even harder to maintain poor body balance and equilibrium.

The Worst Offenders

In Pictures 46 and 47, Kathy and I demonstrate the two most common examples of bad posture. Conscious thought combined with exercise can correct these. In order to develop good posture you must think of the position of your pelvis and your torso in relation to your legs and head, and thinking about your torso helps you to trim it and keep it trimmed. This is why I have included good posture in More Trimming Tips.

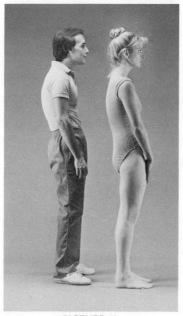

PICTURE 46

Picture 46 depicts the type of posture common in persons who, when carrying a heavy object or even just a carrying case or bag, let the back do most of the work. People who do manual work while standing also have these features prominent. Aside from the reasons previously stated, this kind of postural habit comes from the lack of knowledge and misuse of the torso's units as means of support. Anyone with this type of posture is a sure candidate for back ailments of the worst kind, not to mention circulatory problems such as varicose veins.

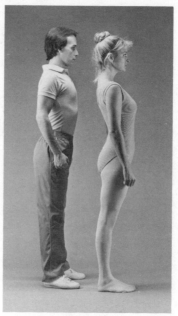

PICTURE 47

Picture 47 is a good example of the old belief, still taught in too many schools, that you should stand with the chest out and the arms back. This position brings undue stress to the lower back and promotes often irreparable weakness in the stomach muscles. Again, learning how to control both of these examples of common bad posture is real simple. But it takes thought in addition to exercise.

Practice Makes Perfect

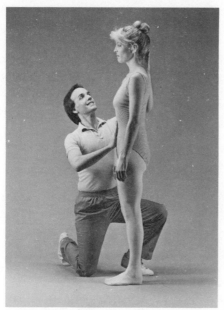

PICTURE 48

Notice how, in Picture 48, I am placing one arm on the center of Kathy's back and one hand on her stomach with fingers pointing toward her head. I am doing this so that she can move her chin straight back until the back of her head touches my hand. This brings the head into alignment with the spine. The fingers of the lower hand are placed upward to indicate to you that the easiest way to sense proper postural alignment is to feel a constant flow of energy that starts from the pelvis and travels upward.

The distribution of your body's weight should be felt in front of the center of the feet and never toward the heels.

The pelvis should never be held in a forced, tucked position and the chest and shoulders should always be kept relaxed and not held.

If you were to hang a plumb line from the ears it should fall slightly in front of the hip bones and end up slightly in front of the center of the feet. Try practicing good postural alignment a few times during your day, and with the help of a stronger torso you will soon have to buy that oversized address book.

Making a Happy Picture

You don't have to wait until you have taken inches off your torso to have the look that comes with good posture. Here's an image exercise that I find works wonders from the first day.

The Champagne Glass: Think of your pelvis as the bowl of a champagne glass that is filled to the rim. The stem of the glass represents your legs and the base your feet. Picture how the bubbles are always moving up. That is the feeling of constant tallness that I spoke of earlier. Visualize how, as you stand, you are carefully balancing the glass so as not to spill a drop. It works. Happy New Posture!

WALKING TALL

Now that your torso has strengthened and trimmed and you have started to consciously think of your posture, it's time to show off. Go for a nice walk and enjoy those looks of jealously and admiration. Look relaxed but don't let go of that feeling of inner strength and natural tallness. Keep that champagne glass filled and bubbly.

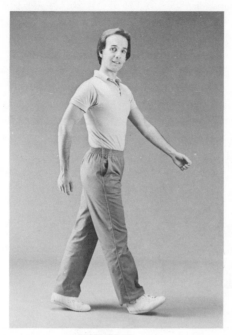

PICTURE 49

Don't let your legs pull you into a walk. Feel as if your newly trimmed torso is rolling on skates. Don't let your weight stay behind. When you walk, feel as if your torso and your front foot reach their destination at the same time. Let the weight roll easily from the heels, over to the balls of the feet as if you were always standing between the front heel and the back toe (Picture 49). Let your arms move in natural opposition to your feet. Hold that head high and smile. A trimmer torso is yours and so is the world. Good hunting. Enjoy it!